Dummies type 2 diabetes diet plan

The Ultimate Guide to Managing Diabetes with a healthy meal plan diet

Dr. Stephen Campbell

Table of contents

INTRODUCTIO

A Journey Back to Health

In the heart of a bustling city, Dr. Stephen Campbell, renowned endocrinologist and diabetes specialist, found himself facing a personal crisis. Despite his expertise in treating type 2 diabetes in his patients, he was blindsided by his own diagnosis. The news hit him like a ton of bricks, shaking him to his core and forcing him to confront his mortality in a way he never imagined.

As Dr. Campbell grappled with the reality of his diagnosis, he was overwhelmed by a whirlwind of emotions-fear, anger, and uncertainty clouded his mind. How could someone who dedicated his life to helping others manage their diabetes find himself in this position? It felt like a cruel twist of fate, a reminder of the fragility of life and the unpredictability of disease.

But amidst the darkness, a flicker of hope emerged. Dr. Campbell refused to let his diagnosis define him. With a steely determination born from years of medical training and a deep-seated desire to reclaim his health, he embarked on a journey of self-discovery and healing.

Drawing upon his expertise as a diabetes specialist, Dr. Campbell dove headfirst into the world of nutrition and lifestyle medicine. He devoured research papers, consulted with fellow experts, and experimented with different dietary approaches, determined to find a solution that would work for him.

As he navigated the ups and downs of his journey, Dr. Campbell experienced firsthand the challenges that his patients faced on a daily basis. He wrestled with cravings, struggled to resist temptation, and grappled with feelings of frustration and self-doubt. But with each setback, he emerged stronger and more determined than ever to succeed.

Slowly but surely, Dr. Campbell began to see progress. His blood sugar levels stabilized, his energy levels soared, and the weight began to melt away. As he reclaimed control of his health, he was filled with a sense of gratitude and humility, humbled by the resilience of the human spirit and the power of healing.

Today, as Dr. Campbell looks back on his journey, he is filled with a profound sense of gratitude. His diagnosis may have been a wake-up call, but it was also a gift—a chance to rediscover what truly matters in life and to inspire others to take charge of their health.

Through his own experience, Dr. Campbell has learned that there is no one-size-fits-all solution to managing type 2 diabetes. But by arming themselves with knowledge, embracing a healthy lifestyle, and never giving up hope, anyone can overcome the challenges of living with diabetes and thrive against all odds.

As the author of "Dummies Type 2 Diabetes Diet Plan," Dr. Campbell invites readers to join him on a journey of transformation, a journey back to health, happiness, and a life lived to the fullest. It's a journey filled with ups and downs, triumphs and setbacks, but above all, it's a journey worth taking.

Defining Diabetes

Diabetes is a chronic metabolic disorder characterized by elevated blood sugar levels due to either insufficient insulin production, resistance to insulin's effects, or a combination of both. Insulin, produced by the pancreas, is a hormone responsible for regulating blood sugar levels and facilitating the uptake of glucose into cells for energy. When this process is disrupted, it leads to hyperglycemia, the hallmark of diabetes.

Looking at Different Types of Diabetes

There are several types of diabetes, with type 1 and type 2 being the most prevalent. Type 1 diabetes, often diagnosed in childhood or adolescence, results from the immune system mistakenly attacking and destroying insulin-producing beta cells in the pancreas. Conversely, type 2 diabetes typically develops in adulthood and is characterized by insulin resistance, where cells fail to respond effectively to insulin. Other less common types include gestational diabetes, which occurs during pregnancy, and monogenic diabetes, resulting from genetic mutations affecting insulin production or function.

Understanding How Diabetes is Diagnosed

Diagnosing diabetes involves assessing blood sugar levels through various tests. The criteria for diagnosing diabetes include:

- Fasting Plasma Glucose Test: A fasting blood sugar level of 126 milligrams per deciliter (mg/dL) or higher indicates diabetes.
- Oral Glucose Tolerance Test (OGTT): A blood sugar level of 200 mg/dL or higher two hours after consuming a glucose solution confirms diabetes.
- Hemoglobin A1c Test: An A1c level of 6.5% or higher reflects long-term blood sugar control and is indicative of diabetes.

Additionally, symptoms such as frequent urination, excessive thirst, unexplained weight loss, and fatigue may prompt further testing for diabetes.

Knowing the Risk Factors

Several factors increase the risk of developing type 2 diabetes, including:

- Obesity or being overweight, especially with excess abdominal fat
- Physical inactivity
- Family history of diabetes
- Age (risk increases with age, particularly after 45)
- Race and ethnicity (higher risk among African Americans, Hispanics, Native Americans, and Asian Americans)
- Gestational diabetes during previous pregnancies
- Polycystic ovary syndrome (PCOS)
- High blood pressure and high cholesterol levels

Understanding these risk factors can aid in early detection and prevention efforts.

Seeing Who Else Has Diabetes

Diabetes is a prevalent condition affecting millions of people worldwide. By exploring statistics and demographics, we can gain insight into the prevalence and distribution of diabetes across different populations. Additionally, sharing personal stories and experiences of individuals living with diabetes can provide valuable perspective and encouragement for those navigating similar challenges.

In the United States alone, over 34 million people have diabetes, with approximately 90-95% diagnosed with type 2 diabetes. This number continues to rise, driven by factors such as aging populations, increasing obesity rates, and sedentary lifestyles. Globally, the World Health Organization (WHO) estimates that over 400 million adults live with diabetes, and this number is projected to surpass 700 million by 2045 if current trends persist.

Diabetes does not discriminate and can affect individuals of all ages, genders, races, and socioeconomic backgrounds. However, certain groups are disproportionately affected. For example, African Americans, Hispanic/Latino Americans, Native Americans, and Asian Americans are at higher risk of developing type 2 diabetes compared to Caucasians. Socioeconomic factors, such as limited access to healthcare and healthy food options, also contribute to disparities in diabetes prevalence and outcomes.

Understanding the diverse populations affected by diabetes is essential for implementing targeted prevention and management strategies. By addressing underlying social determinants of health, promoting lifestyle modifications, and ensuring access to quality healthcare, we can work towards reducing the burden of diabetes and improving the health outcomes of affected individuals and communities.

Why, When, and How to Check Your Blood Glucose

Checking your blood glucose levels is an essential part of managing type 2 diabetes. Here's why, when, and how to monitor your blood glucose effectively:

Why Check Your Blood Glucose:
- Monitoring blood glucose levels helps you understand how your body responds to food, physical activity, medications, and other factors.
- It allows you to make informed decisions about your diet, exercise, and medication regimen to maintain optimal blood sugar control.
- Regular blood glucose monitoring can help identify trends and patterns in your blood sugar levels, enabling you to adjust your

treatment plan accordingly and prevent complications.

When to Check Your Blood Glucose:
- Before meals: Checking your blood glucose before meals helps you determine your baseline blood sugar level and make decisions about mealtime insulin doses or medication adjustments.
- After meals: Checking your blood glucose after meals allows you to see how different foods affect your blood sugar levels and adjust your dietary choices accordingly.
- Before and after exercise: Monitoring blood glucose levels before and after exercise helps you understand how physical activity impacts your blood sugar levels and make adjustments to prevent hypoglycemia (low blood sugar) or hyperglycemia (high blood sugar).
- During illness or stress: During times of illness or stress, blood glucose levels may fluctuate unpredictably. Checking your blood glucose more frequently during these times can help you manage your condition and prevent complications.

How to Check Your Blood Glucose:

- Wash your hands with soap and water and dry them thoroughly.
- Prepare your glucose meter by inserting a test strip into the meter as instructed.
- Use a lancet device to prick the side of your fingertip and collect a small drop of blood.
- Apply the blood sample to the test strip and wait for the meter to display your blood glucose reading.
- Record your blood glucose reading in a logbook or smartphone app to track your progress over time.
- Dispose of used lancets and test strips properly and wash your hands again.

It's important to follow the instructions provided with your glucose meter and test strips carefully to ensure accurate results. Consult your healthcare provider for guidance on how often to check your blood glucose and what target ranges to aim for based on your individual health status and treatment plan.

Chapter 2: The Role of Diet in Managing Type 2 Diabetes

Diet plays a crucial role in managing type 2 diabetes, as it directly impacts blood sugar levels, insulin sensitivity, and overall health. In this chapter, we will explore how dietary choices can influence diabetes management and provide practical guidance for designing a balanced and effective meal plan.

Understanding the Impact of Diet on Blood Sugar Levels

The foods we eat are broken down into glucose, the primary source of energy for our cells. For individuals with type 2 diabetes, the body's ability to regulate blood sugar levels is impaired, leading to elevated glucose levels in the bloodstream. Certain foods, particularly those high in carbohydrates, can cause rapid spikes in blood sugar levels, exacerbating insulin resistance and increasing the risk of complications.

The Importance of Carbohydrate Management

Carbohydrates have the most significant impact on blood sugar levels and should be carefully monitored in the type 2 diabetes diet. Not all carbohydrates are created equal, however. Complex carbohydrates, such as whole grains, fruits, and vegetables, are digested more slowly and have a gentler effect on blood sugar levels compared to simple carbohydrates found in sugary snacks and processed foods. Balancing carbohydrate intake and choosing high-fiber, nutrient-dense options can help stabilize blood sugar levels and improve overall glycemic control.

Prioritizing Protein and Healthy Fats

In addition to carbohydrates, protein and fats also play important roles in the type 2 diabetes diet. Protein helps regulate blood sugar levels and promotes satiety, while healthy fats provide essential nutrients and support heart health. Incorporating lean sources of protein, such as poultry, fish, tofu, and legumes, as well as unsaturated fats from sources like avocados, nuts, and olive oil, can help balance meals and promote better blood sugar management.

Creating a Balanced Meal Plan

A well-balanced meal plan for type 2 diabetes should include a variety of nutrient-rich foods from all food groups. This includes:

- Lean proteins: Chicken, fish, tofu, beans, lentils
- Non-starchy vegetables: Leafy greens, broccoli, peppers, carrots
- Whole grains: Brown rice, quinoa, oats, whole wheat bread
- Healthy fats: Avocado, nuts, seeds, olive oil
- Fruits: Berries, citrus fruits, apples, pears
- Dairy or dairy alternatives: Greek yogurt, almond milk, cottage cheese

Monitoring and Adjusting

Regular monitoring of blood sugar levels is essential for evaluating the effectiveness of dietary interventions and making necessary adjustments. Keeping a food diary, tracking carbohydrate intake, and working with a healthcare provider or registered dietitian can help individuals fine-tune their meal plans to achieve optimal glycemic control and improve long-term outcomes.

The Role of Physical Activity

In addition to diet, regular physical activity is a cornerstone of type 2 diabetes management. Exercise helps improve insulin sensitivity, lower blood sugar levels, and reduce the risk of cardiovascular complications. Incorporating a combination of aerobic exercise, such as walking, cycling, or swimming, and strength training exercises can help individuals with type 2 diabetes achieve and maintain a healthy weight, control blood sugar levels, and improve overall fitness.

Meal Timing and Portion Control

Timing meals and controlling portion sizes are also important aspects of managing type 2 diabetes. Eating regular, balanced meals throughout the day can help stabilize blood sugar levels and prevent spikes and crashes. Additionally, portion control can help individuals manage calorie intake and maintain a healthy weight, which is essential for diabetes management. Using tools such as measuring cups, food scales, and visual cues can help individuals gauge appropriate portion sizes and avoid overeating.

Strategies for Dining Out

Eating away from home presents unique challenges for individuals with type 2 diabetes, as restaurant meals often contain hidden sugars, large portion sizes, and high levels of sodium and unhealthy fats. However, with careful planning and mindful choices, dining out can still be enjoyable and diabetes-friendly. Strategies such as reviewing menus ahead of time, choosing restaurants that offer healthy options, and requesting modifications to dishes can help individuals make healthier choices while dining out.

Overcoming Common Challenges

Living with type 2 diabetes can present various challenges, from managing cravings and dealing with social situations to coping with stress and navigating holidays and special occasions. In this section, we will explore practical tips and strategies for overcoming these common challenges and staying on track with diabetes management. From mindful eating techniques and stress-reduction strategies to meal planning and seeking support from healthcare professionals and peer groups, there are many resources available to help individuals overcome obstacles and achieve long-term success in managing type 2 diabetes.

Setting Realistic Goals and Staying Motivated

Setting realistic goals and staying motivated are key components of successful diabetes management. By setting achievable targets for blood sugar control, weight management, physical activity, and dietary changes, individuals can track their progress and celebrate their successes along the way. Additionally, finding sources of motivation and support, whether it's through personal goals, social connections, or professional guidance, can help individuals stay focused and committed to their diabetes management plan.

Chapter 3: Building a Foundation: Basics of a Type 2 Diabetes Diet

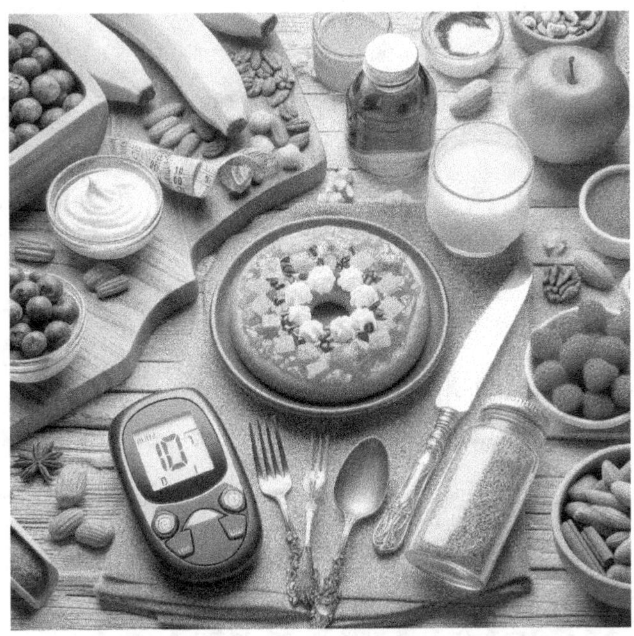

Establishing a strong foundation is essential for effectively managing type 2 diabetes through diet. In this chapter, we will lay out the fundamental principles of a type 2 diabetes diet, providing readers with the knowledge and tools they need to make informed dietary choices and improve their health outcomes.

Emphasizing Whole, Nutrient-Dense Foods

The cornerstone of a type 2 diabetes diet is whole, nutrient-dense foods that provide essential vitamins, minerals, fiber, and antioxidants without excessive added sugars, refined carbohydrates, and unhealthy fats. Examples of nutrient-dense foods include:

- Non-starchy vegetables: Leafy greens, broccoli, cauliflower, bell peppers
- Whole grains: Brown rice, quinoa, oats, barley
- Lean proteins: Chicken, turkey, fish, tofu, beans, lentils
- Healthy fats: Avocado, nuts, seeds, olive oil, fatty fish (salmon, mackerel, sardines)

Monitoring Carbohydrate Intake

Carbohydrates have the most significant impact on blood sugar levels and should be carefully monitored in the type 2 diabetes diet. While carbohydrates are an essential source of energy, not all carbs are created equal. Complex carbohydrates, found in whole grains, fruits, and vegetables, are digested more slowly and have a gentler effect on blood sugar levels compared to simple carbohydrates found in sugary snacks and processed foods.

Incorporating Protein for Satiety and Blood Sugar Control

Protein plays a crucial role in the type 2 diabetes diet, helping regulate blood sugar levels, promote satiety, and support muscle health. Including lean sources of protein such as poultry, fish, tofu, and legumes in meals and snacks can help individuals feel full and satisfied while stabilizing blood sugar levels throughout the day. Additionally, protein-rich foods can be beneficial for weight management and muscle maintenance, both of which are important considerations for individuals with type 2 diabetes.

Balancing Meals and Snacks

Balancing meals and snacks is key to maintaining stable blood sugar levels and avoiding spikes and crashes throughout the day. Aim to include a mix of carbohydrates, protein, and healthy fats in each meal and snack to promote satiety, support blood sugar control, and provide sustained energy. Experiment with different meal combinations and portion sizes to find what works best for your individual needs and preferences.

Hydration and Beverage Choices

Staying hydrated is essential for overall health and wellbeing, particularly for individuals with type 2 diabetes. Water is the best choice for hydration, as it contains no calories or added sugars and helps support optimal bodily functions. Limiting sugary beverages such as soda, fruit juice, and sweetened teas can help reduce unnecessary calorie and sugar intake while promoting better hydration. Opt for water, sparkling water, herbal teas, or unsweetened beverages instead to quench your thirst and support your diabetes management goals.

Planning and Preparing Balanced Meals

Effective meal planning and preparation are essential components of a successful type 2 diabetes diet. By taking the time to plan balanced meals ahead of time and prepare them at home, individuals can ensure they have healthy options readily available and reduce the temptation to rely on convenience foods or takeout.

Consider dedicating time each week to meal planning, grocery shopping, and meal prepping to set yourself up for success. Experiment with new recipes, batch cooking, and meal prepping techniques to streamline the process and make healthy eating more convenient and enjoyable.

Mindful Eating Practices

Practicing mindful eating can help individuals with type 2 diabetes develop a healthier relationship with food and improve their eating habits. Mindful eating involves paying attention to hunger and fullness cues, savoring each bite, and being present and mindful during meals. By slowing down and tuning into your body's signals, you can better regulate portion sizes, reduce overeating, and enhance the overall dining experience. Additionally, mindfulness techniques such as deep breathing, meditation, and journaling can help reduce stress and emotional eating, both of which can impact blood sugar levels and overall health.

Incorporating Flexibility and Variety

While consistency is important for managing blood sugar levels, it's also essential to incorporate flexibility and variety into the type 2 diabetes diet. Strive for balance and moderation rather than strict adherence to rigid rules or restrictions. Allow yourself the flexibility to enjoy occasional treats or indulgences in moderation while staying mindful of portion sizes and overall carbohydrate intake. Additionally, aim to incorporate a wide variety of foods from all food groups to ensure you're getting a diverse range of nutrients and flavors in your diet.

Seeking Support and Accountability

Managing type 2 diabetes can feel overwhelming at times, but you don't have to do it alone. Seeking support and accountability from healthcare professionals, friends, family members, or support groups can provide valuable encouragement, guidance, and motivation along the way. Consider joining a diabetes education program, attending support group meetings, or working with a registered dietitian or certified diabetes educator to develop personalized strategies for success. Building a strong support network can help you stay motivated, overcome challenges, and achieve your health goals.

Monitoring Progress and Adjusting as Needed

Finally, it's essential to monitor your progress regularly and adjust your approach as needed to ensure continued success in managing type 2 diabetes through diet. Keep track of your blood sugar levels, weight, dietary intake, and other relevant metrics to evaluate your progress over time. If you notice any trends or patterns, such as consistently high or low blood sugar levels, consider making adjustments to your meal plan, exercise routine, or medication regimen in collaboration with your healthcare team. By staying proactive and responsive to changes in your health status, you can optimize your diabetes management and improve your overall quality of life.

Thank you for choosing to purchase the "Dummies Type 2 Diabetes Diet Plan" book! Your decision to invest in your health and well-being is truly commendable. As an independent publisher, your support means the world to me, and I'm grateful for the opportunity to share valuable information that can positively impact your life.

Your feedback is incredibly valuable and helps me continue to improve the quality of my publications. If you found the "Dummies Type 2 Diabetes Diet Plan" book helpful, I would greatly appreciate it if you could take a moment to leave a review or share your thoughts. Your feedback not only assists me in refining future editions but also provides valuable insights for other individuals seeking reliable resources for managing type 2 diabetes.

Thank you once again for your support, and I hope the information provided in this book empowers you on your journey to better health and diabetes management.

Chapter 4: Creating Your Type 2 Diabetes Meal Plan

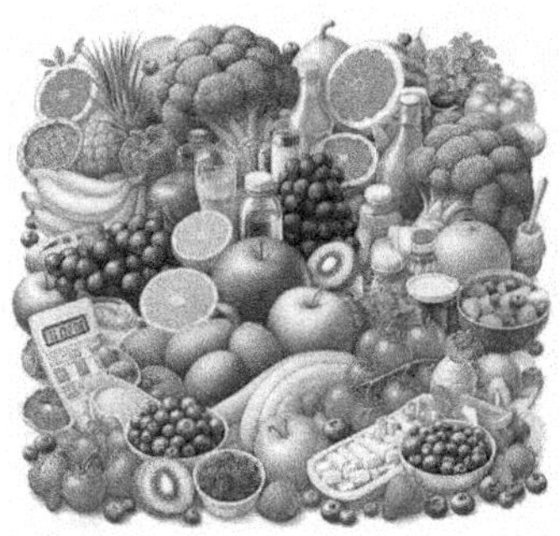

Meal planning is a critical component of effectively managing type 2 diabetes. By carefully selecting and preparing meals ahead of time, individuals with diabetes can better control their blood sugar levels, optimize their nutrient intake, and support their overall health and well-being. Planning meals allows for balanced nutrition, portion control, and consistency, helping to regulate blood sugar levels throughout the day. Additionally, meal planning can reduce the reliance on convenience foods and unhealthy options, making it easier to stick to a diabetes-friendly diet. Overall, meal planning empowers individuals with type 2 diabetes to make informed choices about their dietary intake and take proactive steps towards achieving better health outcomes.

Considering Your Goals of Healthy Eating

When considering your goals for healthy eating while managing type 2 diabetes, it's important to reflect on your individual priorities and aspirations. Healthy eating is not just about controlling blood sugar levels; it's also about nourishing your body, preventing complications, and improving overall well-being. Some personal goals to consider may include:

- Achieving stable blood sugar levels to prevent spikes and crashes throughout the day.
- Managing or achieving a healthy weight to reduce the risk of diabetes-related complications.
- Improving energy levels and reducing fatigue through balanced nutrition.
- Enhancing overall health by incorporating more nutrient-dense foods into your diet.
- Learning to enjoy and appreciate a variety of healthy foods while still indulging in moderation.

Eating Wholesome and Nutritious Food

A key principle of a type 2 diabetes meal plan is prioritizing wholesome, nutrient-dense foods that provide essential vitamins, minerals, fiber, and antioxidants without excess added sugars, refined carbohydrates, and unhealthy fats. Choose a variety of colorful fruits and vegetables, whole grains, lean proteins, and healthy fats to ensure you're getting a diverse range of nutrients and flavors in your diet. Aim to minimize processed and packaged foods, which are often high in sodium, sugar, and unhealthy additives.

Expanding the Selection of Your Food

Expanding your food selection can help keep your meals interesting and enjoyable while ensuring you're getting a wide variety of nutrients in your diet. Experiment with new fruits, vegetables, whole grains, and protein sources to add variety to your meals and snacks. Visit local farmers' markets, ethnic grocery stores, and specialty food shops to discover unique and flavorful ingredients that can spice up your meals and inspire culinary creativity.

Knowing What Counts as One Serving

Understanding serving sizes is essential for portion control and managing carbohydrate intake, particularly for individuals with type 2 diabetes. Familiarize yourself with standard serving sizes for different food groups, such as:

- 1 slice of bread
- 1/2 cup of cooked rice, pasta, or cereal
- 1 cup of raw leafy greens or non-starchy vegetables
- 3 ounces of cooked meat, poultry, or fish
- 1/4 cup of nuts or seeds
- 1 piece of fresh fruit or 1/2 cup of fruit juice

By knowing what counts as one serving, you can better manage your portion sizes and make informed choices about your dietary intake.

Weighing and Measuring Food

To accurately track your food intake and portion sizes, consider investing in a kitchen scale and measuring cups and spoons. Weighing and measuring your food allows you to quantify your portion sizes and ensure you're staying within your recommended carbohydrate, protein, and fat targets. Use these tools regularly, especially when preparing new recipes or foods with unfamiliar portion sizes, to maintain consistency and accuracy in your meal planning.

Knowing How to Create Your Plate

A simple and effective way to build balanced meals is to use the plate method, which divides your plate into specific proportions for different food groups. Aim to fill half your plate with non-starchy vegetables, one-quarter with lean protein, and one-quarter with whole grains or starchy vegetables. Add a serving of fruit and a small portion of healthy fats to round out your meal. This approach helps ensure you're getting a variety of nutrients while controlling portion sizes and managing blood sugar levels.

Meal Plans That Work for You

When creating your meal plan, consider your lifestyle, preferences, and dietary restrictions to develop a plan that works for you. Some individuals may prefer structured meal plans with specific recipes and portion sizes, while others may prefer a more flexible approach with guidelines and suggestions for meal components. Experiment with different meal planning strategies, such as batch cooking, meal prepping, or intuitive eating, to find what works best for your schedule, tastes, and health goals.

Chapter 5 : Introduction to Carbohydrate Counting

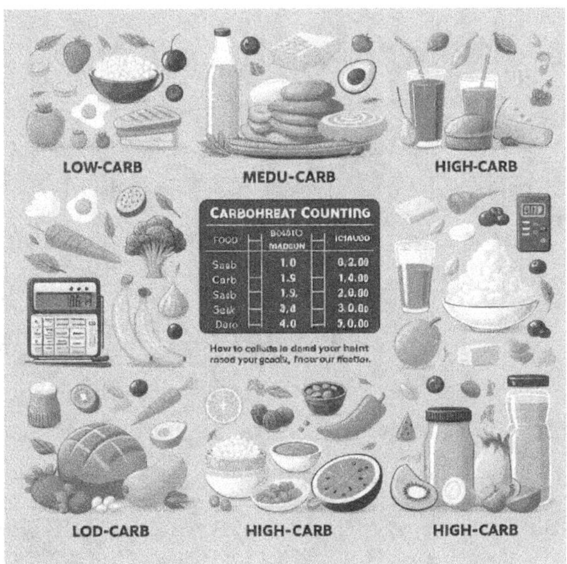

Carbohydrate counting is a valuable tool for individuals with type 2 diabetes to manage their blood sugar levels and insulin dosing. By accurately counting the carbohydrates in your meals and snacks, you can better regulate your blood sugar levels and make informed decisions about your dietary intake. Learn how to identify sources of carbohydrates in your diet, read nutrition labels, and estimate portion sizes to calculate your carbohydrate intake accurately.

Working with a registered dietitian or certified diabetes educator can help you learn the basics of carbohydrate counting and develop a personalized plan that meets your individual needs and goals.

Best carbohydrates diet for type 2 diabetes

A well-balanced carbohydrate diet for individuals with type 2 diabetes focuses on consuming carbohydrates that have a low glycemic index (GI) and are high in fiber. These carbohydrates are beneficial for managing blood sugar levels because they are digested and absorbed more slowly, resulting in gradual increases in blood glucose levels and better glycemic control. Here's a sample of the best carbohydrates for type 2 diabetes:

- **Whole grains:**

Examples: Quinoa, brown rice, oats, barley, whole wheat bread, whole grain pasta.

Why they're the best: Whole grains are rich in fiber, vitamins, and minerals. They have a lower glycemic index compared to refined grains, which means they cause a slower and more gradual rise in blood sugar levels after consumption.

Carb count: A 1/2 cup serving of cooked quinoa contains approximately 20 grams of carbohydrates.

• Legumes:

Examples: Lentils, chickpeas, black beans, kidney beans, edamame.

Why they're the best: Legumes are high in fiber and protein, which help stabilize blood sugar levels and promote feelings of fullness. They also contain resistant starch, a type of carbohydrate that is not fully digested and may have beneficial effects on blood sugar control.

Carb count: A 1/2 cup serving of cooked lentils contains approximately 20 grams of carbohydrates.

• Non-starchy vegetables:

Examples: Leafy greens (spinach, kale, lettuce), broccoli, cauliflower, bell peppers, cucumbers, zucchini.

Why they're the best: Non-starchy vegetables are low in carbohydrates and calories but high in fiber, vitamins, and minerals. They have a minimal impact on blood sugar levels and can be eaten in large quantities without significantly affecting blood glucose.

Carb count: A 1/2 cup serving of cooked broccoli contains approximately 3 grams of carbohydrates.

- **Fruits:**

Examples: Berries (strawberries, blueberries, raspberries), apples, oranges, pears, kiwi.

Why they're the best: Fruits are natural sources of carbohydrates, but they also contain fiber, vitamins, and antioxidants, which help slow down the absorption of sugar into the bloodstream. Berries, in particular, have a lower glycemic index compared to other fruits.

Carb count: A small apple contains approximately 15 grams of carbohydrates.

- **Nuts and seeds:**

Examples: Almonds, walnuts, chia seeds, flaxseeds, pumpkin seeds.

Why they're the best: Nuts and seeds are rich in healthy fats, protein, and fiber, which help stabilize blood sugar levels and promote satiety. They are low in carbohydrates and can be included as part of a balanced diet for individuals with type 2 diabetes.

Carb count: A 1-ounce serving of almonds contains approximately 6 grams of carbohydrates.

It's important to note that portion control is key when including carbohydrates in a diabetes diet. While these carbohydrates are considered "better" choices for managing blood sugar levels, moderation is still important to prevent spikes in blood glucose. Consulting with a registered dietitian or healthcare provider can help tailor a carbohydrate diet plan that meets individual needs and supports optimal diabetes management.

Worse carbohydrates diet for type 2 diabetes

A diet high in refined carbohydrates and added sugars is considered worse for individuals with type 2 diabetes. These carbohydrates have a high glycemic index (GI), meaning they are quickly digested and absorbed, causing rapid spikes in blood sugar levels. Here's a sample of the worst carbohydrates for type 2 diabetes:

- **Refined grains:**

Examples: White bread, white rice, white pasta, pastries, sugary cereals.

Why they're the worst: Refined grains have been processed to remove the bran and germ, stripping away most of the fiber, vitamins, and minerals. They are quickly broken down into sugar in the body, leading to rapid increases in blood glucose levels.

Carb count: A 1-ounce slice of white bread contains approximately 15 grams of carbohydrates.

- **Sugary beverages:**

Examples: Soda, fruit juice, sweetened iced tea, energy drinks.

Why they're the worst: Sugary beverages are loaded with added sugars and provide empty calories with little to no nutritional value. They cause rapid spikes in blood sugar levels and can contribute to weight gain, insulin resistance, and poor blood sugar control.

Carb count: A 12-ounce can of soda contains approximately 40 grams of carbohydrates.

• **Processed snacks and sweets:**

Examples: Candy, cookies, cakes, chips, crackers, sweetened yogurt.

Why they're the worst: Processed snacks and sweets are typically high in refined carbohydrates, added sugars, unhealthy fats, and sodium. They provide little satiety and can lead to overeating, weight gain, and unstable blood sugar levels.

Carb count: A single chocolate chip cookie contains approximately 15 grams of carbohydrates.

• **Sugary breakfast cereals:**

Examples: Frosted flakes, Froot Loops, Cocoa Puffs, sugary granola.

Why they're the worst: Breakfast cereals marketed to children are often high in sugar and low in fiber, providing a quick energy boost followed by a crash in blood sugar levels. They lack nutritional value and can contribute to insulin resistance and obesity.

Carb count: A 1-cup serving of sugary breakfast cereal can contain 30 grams or more of carbohydrates.

• **Processed and sugary sauces:**

Examples: Barbecue sauce, ketchup, sweet chili sauce, teriyaki sauce.

Why they're the worst: Processed sauces and condiments are often high in added sugars, hidden carbohydrates, and unhealthy additives. They can significantly increase the carbohydrate content of meals and contribute to elevated blood sugar levels.

Carb count: A tablespoon of barbecue sauce can contain approximately 10 grams of carbohydrates.

These worst carbohydrates for type 2 diabetes should be limited or avoided in the diet to maintain stable blood sugar levels, support weight management, and reduce the risk of diabetes-related complications. Choosing whole, minimally processed foods and beverages that are lower in added sugars and higher in fiber is key to achieving better blood sugar control and overall health.

Planning Smart:

Meal planning is a key strategy for successfully managing type 2 diabetes and achieving your health goals. Here are some effective strategies for planning your meals:

Set aside time: Dedicate a specific time each week to plan your meals. This could be a Sunday afternoon or any other day that works best for you. Use this time to review your schedule for the upcoming week, consider any special occasions or events, and plan your meals accordingly.

Consider personal preferences: Take into account your personal food preferences, dietary restrictions, and cultural or culinary traditions when planning your meals. Choose recipes and ingredients that you enjoy and that align with your taste preferences and health goals.

Create a shopping list: Once you've planned your meals for the week, create a shopping list of all the ingredients you'll need. Organize your list by food categories (e.g., fruits and vegetables, protein sources, pantry staples) to make shopping more efficient and ensure you don't forget anything. Check your pantry and refrigerator to see what items you already have on hand and only purchase what you need.

Focus on balance: Aim to create balanced meals that include a mix of carbohydrates, protein, and healthy fats. Incorporate a variety of colorful fruits and vegetables, whole grains, lean proteins, and plant-based fats into your meals to ensure you're getting a wide range of nutrients. Consider using tools such as the plate method or the diabetes food pyramid to guide your meal planning and portion sizes.

Batch cooking and meal prep: Consider batch cooking or meal prepping to save time and simplify meal preparation during the week. Cook large batches of grains, proteins, and vegetables ahead of time and portion them out into individual containers for easy grab-and-go meals. Alternatively, prepare ingredients in advance (e.g., chopping vegetables, marinating meats) to streamline cooking during the week.

Be flexible: While meal planning can help provide structure and consistency, it's important to remain flexible and adaptable. Life can be unpredictable, and plans may change, so be prepared to adjust your meal plan as needed. Have backup options available for busy nights or unexpected events, such as quick and easy recipes or healthy convenience foods.

Shopping Smart:

Grocery shopping is a crucial step in implementing a healthy eating plan for managing type 2 diabetes. Here are some tips to help you shop smart and make nutritious choices at the grocery store:

Focus on nutrient-dense foods: Choose foods that are rich in essential nutrients such as vitamins, minerals, fiber, and antioxidants. Prioritize fresh fruits and vegetables, whole grains, lean proteins (such as poultry, fish, tofu, and legumes), and healthy fats (such as avocados, nuts, seeds, and olive oil). These nutrient-dense foods provide valuable nutrition without excess calories, added sugars, or unhealthy fats.

Read labels: Take the time to read nutrition labels carefully when selecting packaged foods. Pay attention to serving sizes, total carbohydrate content (including sugars and fiber), protein, fat, and sodium levels. Look for products with minimal added sugars, trans fats, and sodium, and choose options with higher fiber content to help regulate blood sugar levels and promote satiety.

Plan your meals and make a list: Before heading to the grocery store, plan your meals for the week and make a list of all the ingredients you'll need. Organize your list by food categories to make shopping more efficient and prevent impulse purchases. Stick to your list as much as possible to avoid unnecessary spending and temptation.

Shop the perimeter: The perimeter of the grocery store is typically where you'll find fresh produce, lean proteins, dairy products, and whole grains. Focus on shopping the perimeter first before venturing into the inner aisles, where processed and packaged foods are often located. By prioritizing whole, unprocessed foods, you'll fill your cart with nutrient-dense options that support your health goals.

Avoid shopping when hungry: Shopping on an empty stomach can lead to impulse purchases of unhealthy snacks and convenience foods. Eat a balanced meal or snack before heading to the grocery store to help curb cravings and make healthier choices.

Choose seasonal and local produce: Opt for seasonal fruits and vegetables when possible, as they tend to be fresher, more flavorful, and more affordable. Consider shopping at farmers' markets or joining a community-supported agriculture (CSA) program to access locally grown produce and support local farmers.

Limit processed and packaged foods: Minimize your intake of processed and packaged foods, which are often high in added sugars, unhealthy fats, and sodium. Instead, focus on whole, minimally processed foods that provide essential nutrients and support your overall health and well-being.

7-day grocery shopping list

Here's a sample grocery shopping list for a week of meals:

Produce:

- Spinach or mixed greens
- Broccoli
- Bell peppers (red, green, or yellow)
- Carrots
- Tomatoes
- Onions
- Garlic
- Avocados
- Apples
- Bananas
- Berries (strawberries, blueberries, raspberries)
- Lemons or limes

Protein:
- Chicken breasts or thighs
- Salmon fillets
- Lean ground turkey or beef
- Eggs
- Greek yogurt
- Tofu or tempeh

Grains and Legumes:
- Brown rice
- Quinoa
- Whole wheat pasta or noodles
- Whole grain bread or wraps

- Lentils
- Canned beans (black beans, chickpeas, kidney beans)

Dairy and Alternatives:
- Low-fat milk or unsweetened almond milk
- Cottage cheese
- Cheese (cheddar, mozzarella, feta)
- Plain yogurt (regular or dairy-free)

Nuts, Seeds, and Oils:
- Almonds
- Walnuts
- Chia seeds
- Flaxseeds
- Olive oil
- Coconut oil or avocado oil

Pantry Staples:
- Canned tomatoes (diced or crushed)
- Tomato sauce or marinara sauce (no added sugar)
- Chicken or vegetable broth (low-sodium)
- Spices and herbs (salt-free blends, garlic powder, onion powder, oregano, basil)
- Whole grain cereal or oats

- Whole grain crackers or rice cakes
- Nut butter (peanut butter, almond butter)
- Popcorn kernels

Frozen Foods:
- Frozen mixed vegetables
- Frozen berries
- Frozen shrimp or fish fillets
- Frozen edamame or green peas

This list provides a variety of nutritious ingredients that can be used to prepare balanced meals throughout the week. Adjust quantities based on your individual needs and preferences, and feel free to add any additional items that you enjoy or need for specific recipes. Happy shopping and happy cooking!

Cooking Smart:

Cooking at home is a key component of a healthy lifestyle, especially for individuals managing type 2 diabetes. Here are some cooking techniques and strategies to help you prepare nutritious meals at home efficiently:

Batch cooking: Batch cooking involves preparing large quantities of food at once and portioning it out for multiple meals throughout the week. Choose a day when you have some extra time, such as a weekend day, to cook in bulk. Prepare staple ingredients such as brown rice, quinoa, roasted vegetables, grilled chicken, or lean ground turkey in large batches. Portion them into individual containers or freezer bags and store them in the refrigerator or freezer for easy grab-and-go meals during the week. Batch cooking saves time and ensures you have healthy options readily available when hunger strikes.

Meal prep: Meal prep involves prepping ingredients or assembling meals ahead of time to streamline cooking during the week. Spend some time each week washing, chopping, and portioning out fruits, vegetables, and other ingredients for your meals. Pre-cook grains, proteins, and sauces to have them ready to go when you're ready to cook. Consider assembling make-ahead meals such as salads, stir-fries, or casseroles that can be quickly reheated or finished off when you're short on time. Meal prep helps you stay organized and makes it easier to stick to your healthy eating plan throughout the week.

Use kitchen tools efficiently: Invest in kitchen tools and appliances that make cooking easier and more efficient. A few essential tools to have on hand include a sharp chef's knife, cutting board, vegetable peeler, and can opener. Consider investing in a slow cooker or Instant Pot for hands-off cooking of soups, stews, and one-pot meals. Use kitchen gadgets such as a food processor, blender, or spiralizer to quickly chop, blend, or prep ingredients. Opt for non-stick cookware to reduce the need for excess oil when cooking. By using kitchen tools efficiently, you can save time and effort in the kitchen while still preparing delicious and nutritious meals.

Experiment with cooking techniques: Get creative in the kitchen and experiment with different cooking techniques to add flavor and variety to your meals. Try grilling, baking, roasting, steaming, sautéing, or stir-frying your ingredients to see which methods you prefer. Use herbs, spices, citrus juices, and vinegar to season your dishes without relying on excess salt, sugar, or unhealthy fats. Incorporate healthy cooking fats such as olive oil, avocado oil, or coconut oil for added flavor and richness. By exploring new cooking techniques, you can discover new favorite recipes and make mealtime more enjoyable.

By incorporating batch cooking, meal prep, efficient kitchen tools, and varied cooking techniques into your routine, you can prepare nutritious meals at home with ease. Experiment with different strategies to find what works best for you and your lifestyle, and don't be afraid to get creative in the kitchen. With a little planning and preparation, you can enjoy delicious and healthy meals that support your type 2 diabetes management goals.

Tempting Your Taste Buds with Nutritious Nibbles:

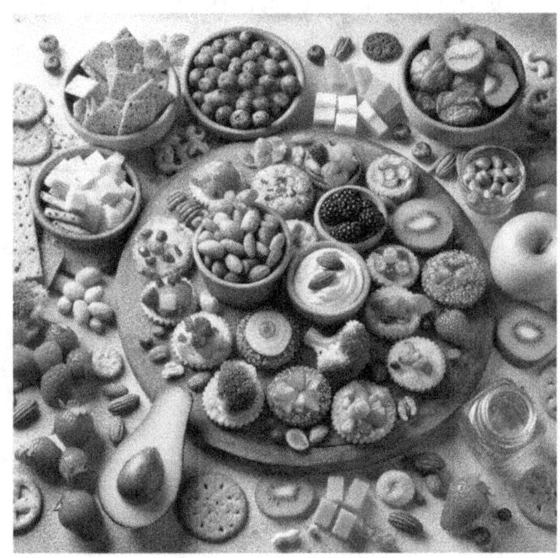

Snacking can be a satisfying and enjoyable part of your type 2 diabetes meal plan, offering opportunities to refuel between meals and satisfy cravings. Here are some snack options categorized by their carbohydrate content, along with strategies for incorporating them into your meal plan:

Low-Carb Options (5 grams of carbs or less per serving):

- Hard-boiled egg: 0 grams of carbs
- Raw vegetables (carrot sticks, cucumber slices, bell pepper strips) with hummus: 5 grams of carbs per 1/4 cup of hummus
- String cheese: 0 grams of carbs
- Greek yogurt with berries: 5 grams of carbs per 1/2 cup of Greek yogurt and 1/4 cup of berries
- Nuts and seeds (almonds, walnuts, pumpkin seeds): 2-4 grams of carbs per 1 ounce serving

Moderate-Carb Options (10-20 grams of carbs per serving):

- Apple slices with almond butter: 15 grams of carbs per medium apple and 1 tablespoon of almond butter

- Cottage cheese with pineapple chunks: 14 grams of carbs per 1/2 cup of cottage cheese and 1/2 cup of pineapple chunks
- Rice cakes with avocado: 14 grams of carbs per rice cake and 1/4 of an avocado
- Edamame: 8 grams of carbs per 1/2 cup serving (shelled)
- Turkey and cheese roll-ups: 6 grams of carbs per 2 slices of turkey and 1 slice of cheese

High-Carb Options (20 grams of carbs or more per serving):

- Whole grain crackers with hummus: 22 grams of carbs per 6 whole grain crackers and 1/4 cup of hummus
- Popcorn: 20 grams of carbs per 3 cups popped
- Trail mix: 25 grams of carbs per 1/4 cup serving
- Banana with peanut butter: 27 grams of carbs per medium banana and 2 tablespoons of peanut butter
- Dried fruit (raisins, apricots, dates): 22-28 grams of carbs per 1/4 cup serving

Strategies for Incorporating Healthy Snacks:

- Plan ahead: Pack snacks in advance so you have them on hand when hunger strikes.
- Portion control: Measure out servings to avoid overeating and maintain blood sugar control.
- Pair carbs with protein or healthy fats: Combining carbohydrates with protein or healthy fats can help stabilize blood sugar levels and keep you feeling full longer.
- Listen to your body: Snack when you're hungry, but pay attention to portion sizes and choose nutrient-dense options.

Experiment with flavors and textures: Try new snack combinations to keep things interesting and satisfy your taste buds.

Eating Out with Confidence

Navigating restaurant menus can be challenging when managing type 2 diabetes, but with the right strategies, you can enjoy dining out while staying on track with your meal plan. Here are some tips for eating out with confidence:

- **Selecting Restaurants with Healthy Choices**

Choose restaurants that offer a variety of healthy options, such as salads, grilled proteins, and vegetable-based dishes. Look for establishments that prioritize fresh, whole ingredients and offer customizable menu options to accommodate dietary preferences and restrictions. Avoid fast food chains and buffets, which tend to offer limited healthy choices and large portion sizes that can make it difficult to control your carbohydrate intake.

- **Ordering Meals that Mesh with Your Plan**

When ordering at a restaurant, opt for dishes that align with your type 2 diabetes meal plan. Start with a lean protein source, such as grilled chicken, fish, or tofu, and pair it with non-starchy vegetables or a side salad. Request dressings and sauces on the side to control portion sizes and minimize added sugars and unhealthy fats. Choose whole grain or vegetable-based options, such as brown rice, quinoa, or cauliflower rice, instead of refined grains like white rice or pasta. Be mindful of portion sizes and consider sharing entrees or asking for a half portion if the serving size is large.

- **Celebrations and Special Occasions**

While special occasions and celebrations often involve indulgent foods and treats, you can still enjoy yourself while managing type 2 diabetes. Plan ahead by checking the restaurant menu online and identifying healthier options that fit within your meal plan. Consider eating a small, balanced meal or snack before the event to help control hunger and prevent overeating. Focus on socializing and enjoying the company of friends and family rather than solely on the food. Practice moderation and portion control, and allow yourself to indulge in small portions of your favorite treats if desired. Remember that one meal or occasional splurge won't derail your progress, but consistency and balance are key to long-term success in managing type 2 diabetes.

Chapter 6 : The Power of Protein in Managing Type 2 Diabetes

Protein plays a crucial role in managing type 2 diabetes and maintaining overall health. This chapter explores the importance of protein in the diet of individuals with type 2 diabetes and how it can positively impact blood sugar control, weight management, and muscle health. Topics covered include the benefits of protein, sources of protein, recommended intake, and strategies for incorporating protein into meals and snacks.

Importance of Protein:

- Protein is essential for building and repairing tissues, including muscles, bones, and organs.
- It plays a key role in regulating blood sugar levels by slowing down the absorption of carbohydrates and promoting satiety, which can help prevent spikes in blood sugar after meals.
- Protein-rich foods tend to have a lower impact on blood sugar levels compared to high-carbohydrate foods, making them a valuable component of a diabetes-friendly diet.

Benefits of Protein:

- **Helps control blood sugar levels**: Protein slows down the absorption of glucose into the bloodstream, preventing rapid spikes and promoting more stable blood sugar levels.
- **Supports weight management**: Protein-rich foods are filling and can help curb appetite, leading to reduced calorie intake and improved weight management.
- **Maintains muscle mass**: Adequate protein intake is essential for preserving muscle mass, especially in individuals with type 2 diabetes who may be at risk of muscle loss due to aging or inactivity.
- **Promotes satiety:** Protein-rich foods are more satisfying and can help control cravings and prevent overeating, leading to better appetite control and weight management.

Sources of Protein:

- **Lean meats:** Skinless poultry, lean cuts of beef or pork, and seafood are excellent sources of protein with minimal saturated fat.

- **Plant-based proteins**: Legumes (such as beans, lentils, and chickpeas), tofu, tempeh, edamame, and quinoa are nutritious plant-based sources of protein.
- **Dairy and dairy alternatives**: Greek yogurt, cottage cheese, milk, and dairy-free alternatives like almond milk and soy milk provide protein along with essential nutrients like calcium and vitamin D.
- **Eggs**: Eggs are a versatile and affordable source of high-quality protein, as well as essential nutrients like vitamins B12 and D.
- **Nuts and seeds**: Almonds, walnuts, peanuts, chia seeds, and hemp seeds are nutrient-dense sources of protein, healthy fats, and fiber.

Recommended Intake:

- The recommended daily intake of protein varies depending on factors such as age, sex, activity level, and overall health status.
- In general, aim to include a source of protein in each meal and snack to support muscle health, blood sugar control, and overall well-being.
- Consult with a healthcare provider or registered dietitian to determine your

individual protein needs and develop a personalized nutrition plan.

Strategies for Incorporating Protein:

- **Include a protein source in each meal and snack**: Pair protein-rich foods with carbohydrates and healthy fats to create balanced meals that support blood sugar control and satiety.

- **Plan ahead**: Batch cook protein-rich foods such as grilled chicken, hard-boiled eggs, or tofu to have on hand for quick and easy meals throughout the week.

- **Experiment with plant-based proteins:** Incorporate more plant-based protein sources into your diet, such as beans, lentils, and soy products, to increase variety and nutrient intake.

- **Choose lean options**: Opt for lean cuts of meat, poultry without skin, and low-fat dairy products to minimize saturated fat intake and support heart health.

Chapter 7: Healthy Fats and Their Impact on Blood Sugar Levels

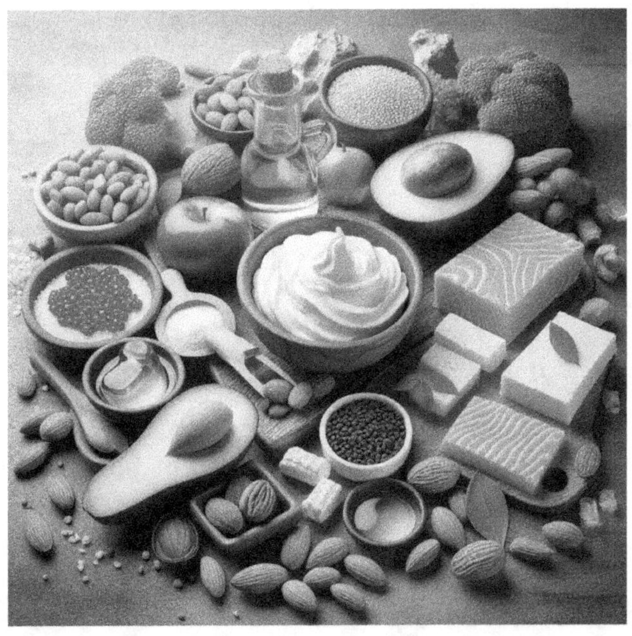

Understanding the role of fats in managing type 2 diabetes is crucial for achieving optimal health outcomes. This chapter explores the impact of healthy fats on blood sugar levels and provides insights into how incorporating the right types of fats into your diet can support blood sugar control, heart health, and overall well-being.

Topics covered include the benefits of healthy fats, sources of healthy fats, recommended intake, and practical tips for incorporating healthy fats into meals and snacks. Readers will gain valuable knowledge on how to make informed choices about fat consumption to improve their diabetes management and overall health.

Importance of Healthy Fats:

- Healthy fats are essential for overall health, including heart health, brain function, and hormone production.
- Unlike saturated and trans fats, healthy fats have been shown to have a neutral or positive effect on blood sugar levels and insulin sensitivity, making them an important component of a diabetes-friendly diet.
- Consuming healthy fats in moderation can help improve blood sugar control, reduce inflammation, and lower the risk of cardiovascular disease, which is common in individuals with type 2 diabetes.

Benefits of Healthy Fats:

- **Supports heart health:** Healthy fats, such as monounsaturated and polyunsaturated fats, can help lower LDL (bad) cholesterol levels and reduce the risk of heart disease.

- **Provides essential nutrients**: Healthy fats are a concentrated source of essential fatty acids, such as omega-3 and omega-6 fatty acids, which are important for brain health, immune function, and inflammation regulation.

- **Promotes satiety:** Including healthy fats in meals and snacks can help increase feelings of fullness and satisfaction, leading to better appetite control and reduced cravings for unhealthy foods.

- **Enhances nutrient absorption**: Fat-soluble vitamins (vitamins A, D, E, and K) require fat for absorption, so consuming healthy fats with meals can help ensure you get the maximum nutritional benefit from your food.

Sources of Healthy Fats:

- **Avocados**: Avocados are rich in monounsaturated fats, which have been linked to improved heart health and blood sugar control.

- **Nuts and seeds**: Almonds, walnuts, flaxseeds, chia seeds, and hemp seeds are excellent sources of healthy fats, protein, and fiber.
- **Olive oil:** Extra virgin olive oil is a staple of the Mediterranean diet and is high in monounsaturated fats, antioxidants, and anti-inflammatory compounds.
- **Fatty fish**: Salmon, mackerel, trout, and sardines are rich in omega-3 fatty acids, which have been shown to reduce inflammation and improve heart health.
- **Nut butters**: Peanut butter, almond butter, and other nut butters are tasty sources of healthy fats and protein that can be enjoyed as spreads or added to smoothies and oatmeal.

Recommended Intake:

- The American Diabetes Association recommends that healthy fats should make up about 20-35% of your total daily calorie intake.
- Aim to include a variety of sources of healthy fats in your diet, such as nuts, seeds, avocados, olive oil, and fatty fish, to ensure you're getting a balanced mix of essential fatty acids and nutrients.

Practical Tips for Incorporating Healthy Fats:

- Use olive oil or avocado oil for cooking and salad dressings instead of butter or margarine.
- Snack on a handful of nuts or seeds for a satisfying and nutritious snack.
- Add avocado slices or nut butter to smoothies, salads, or whole grain toast for extra flavor and healthy fats.
- Choose fatty fish like salmon or trout as the main protein in your meals at least twice a week.
- Be mindful of portion sizes when consuming high-fat foods, as they are calorie-dense and can contribute to weight gain if consumed in excess.

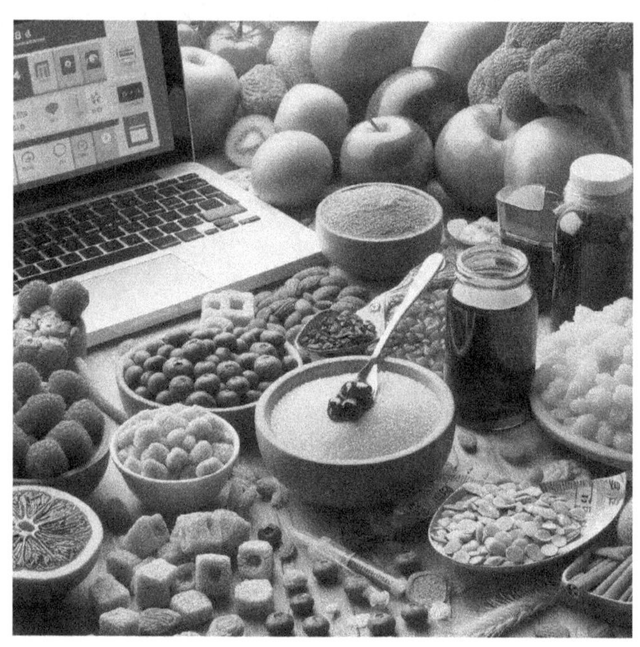

Incorporating Fiber for Better Blood Sugar Management

Chapter 8: Incorporating Fiber for Better Blood Sugar Management

Understanding the role of fiber in managing blood sugar levels is essential for individuals with type 2 diabetes. Here's a breakdown of the information covered in this chapter:

Importance of Fiber:

- Fiber is a type of carbohydrate found in plant-based foods that cannot be digested by the body. Instead, it passes through the digestive system intact, providing numerous health benefits.
- Dietary fiber plays a crucial role in regulating blood sugar levels by slowing down the absorption of glucose into the bloodstream. This helps prevent rapid spikes in blood sugar after meals and promotes more stable blood sugar levels over time.
- Fiber also helps promote satiety, improve digestive health, and reduce the risk of chronic

diseases such as heart disease, obesity, and certain types of cancer.

Benefits of Fiber:

- **Supports blood sugar control**: Fiber-rich foods help regulate blood sugar levels by slowing down the absorption of carbohydrates and preventing sudden spikes in blood glucose after meals.

- **Promotes satiety:** High-fiber foods are more filling and satisfying, leading to reduced hunger and cravings, which can help with weight management and blood sugar control.

- **Improves digestive health**: Fiber adds bulk to stool, promoting regular bowel movements and preventing constipation. It also supports a healthy gut microbiome, which is important for overall digestive health and immune function.

- **Reduces the risk of chronic disease**: Consuming an adequate amount of dietary fiber has been linked to a reduced risk of heart disease, stroke, obesity, and certain types of cancer.

Sources of Fiber:

- **Whole grains**: Whole wheat, oats, barley, quinoa, brown rice, and bulgur are excellent sources of dietary fiber. Choose whole grain options over refined grains to maximize fiber intake.

- **Fruits and vegetables**: Berries, apples, pears, oranges, broccoli, carrots, spinach, and Brussels sprouts are rich in fiber and other essential nutrients. Aim to include a variety of colorful fruits and vegetables in your diet to increase fiber intake.

- **Legumes**: Beans, lentils, chickpeas, and split peas are high in fiber and protein, making them excellent additions to soups, salads, and main dishes.

- **Nuts and seeds**: Almonds, chia seeds, flaxseeds, and sunflower seeds are nutritious sources of fiber, healthy fats, and protein. Enjoy them as snacks or add them to yogurt, oatmeal, or smoothies for an extra fiber boost.

Recommended Intake:

- The American Diabetes Association recommends consuming a minimum of 25-30 grams of fiber per day for adults, with a focus on increasing intake from whole foods rather than supplements.

- Gradually increase fiber intake over time to allow your digestive system to adjust and prevent gastrointestinal discomfort.

Practical Tips for Incorporating Fiber:

- Start your day with a high-fiber breakfast, such as oatmeal topped with fruit and nuts or whole grain toast with avocado.
- Include a serving of fruits or vegetables with every meal and snack to increase fiber intake.
- Choose whole grain options such as brown rice, whole wheat pasta, and whole grain bread over refined grains.
- Snack on fiber-rich foods like raw vegetables with hummus, whole fruit, or air-popped popcorn.
- Experiment with new recipes and ingredients to incorporate more fiber-rich foods into your diet, such as adding beans to soups and salads or using cauliflower rice as a lower-carb alternative to white rice.

Chapter 9: Hydration and Its Importance for Type 2 Diabetics

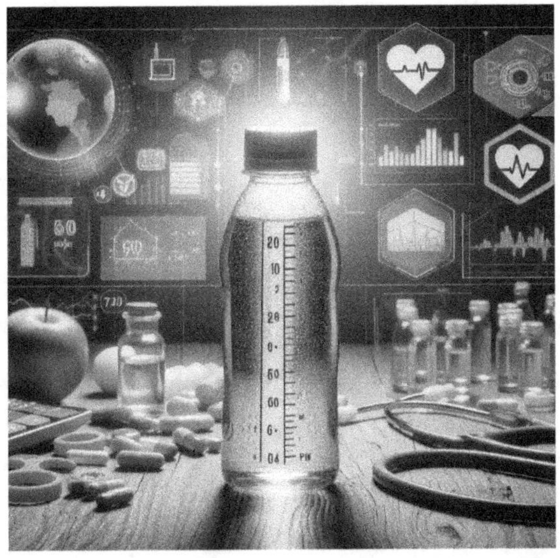

Hydration plays a vital role in overall health and well-being, especially for individuals with type 2 diabetes. This chapter explores the importance of hydration, the impact of dehydration on blood sugar control, and practical strategies for staying properly hydrated. By understanding the significance of hydration and implementing hydration best practices, individuals with type 2 diabetes can support their health and optimize their diabetes management.

Importance of Hydration:

- Hydration is essential for maintaining proper bodily functions, including regulating body temperature, transporting nutrients, and eliminating waste products.
- For individuals with type 2 diabetes, hydration is particularly important because dehydration can exacerbate symptoms and lead to complications such as hyperglycemia (high blood sugar) and diabetic ketoacidosis (DKA).
- Proper hydration supports kidney function, which is crucial for filtering waste products from the blood and maintaining electrolyte balance.

Impact of Dehydration on Blood Sugar Control:

- Dehydration can cause blood sugar levels to become more concentrated, leading to higher blood sugar readings.
- When the body is dehydrated, the kidneys release more glucose into the urine to try to dilute the blood, resulting in increased urination and potential dehydration.

- Dehydration can also affect insulin sensitivity, making it more challenging to control blood sugar levels effectively.

Recommended Hydration Practices:

- **Drink plenty of water**: Aim to drink at least 8-10 cups of water per day, or more if you're physically active or exposed to hot temperatures.

- **Monitor urine color**: Check the color of your urine to assess hydration status. Clear or pale yellow urine indicates adequate hydration, while dark yellow or amber urine may signal dehydration.

- **Spread out water intake**: Drink water consistently throughout the day rather than consuming large amounts at once. Sipping water regularly helps maintain hydration levels and prevents dehydration.

- **Be mindful of other beverages**: While water is the best choice for hydration, other beverages such as herbal tea, unsweetened coffee, and low-calorie flavored water can also contribute to overall fluid intake. Limit consumption of sugary drinks and alcohol, as they can contribute to dehydration and affect blood sugar levels.

Hydration Tips for Type 2 Diabetics:

- **Monitor blood sugar levels**: Keep track of blood sugar readings and hydration status to identify any patterns or correlations between dehydration and blood sugar fluctuations.
- **Adjust insulin or medication doses**: If dehydration leads to higher blood sugar levels, consult with a healthcare provider to adjust insulin or medication doses as needed to maintain blood sugar control.
- **Stay hydrated during exercise:** Drink water before, during, and after exercise to replace fluids lost through sweat. Monitor blood sugar levels more frequently during exercise, as physical activity can affect hydration and blood sugar levels.

Signs of Dehydration:

- Thirst
- Dry mouth and lips

- Dark yellow urine
- Fatigue or weakness
- Dizziness or lightheadedness
- Headache
- Decreased urine output

Proper hydration is essential for individuals with type 2 diabetes to support overall health and blood sugar control. By staying adequately hydrated and monitoring hydration status regularly, individuals can optimize their diabetes management and reduce the risk of dehydration-related complications.

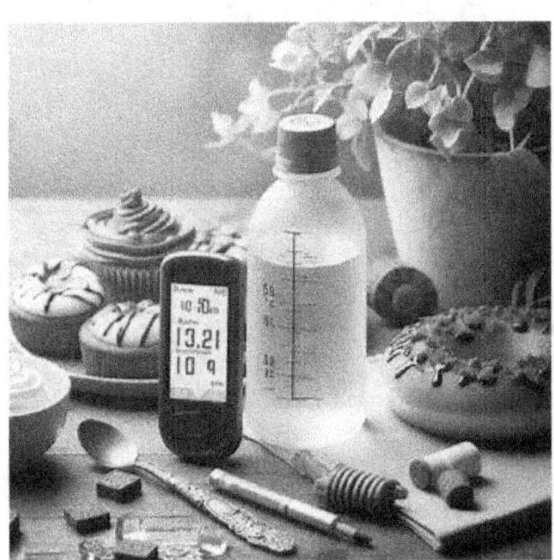

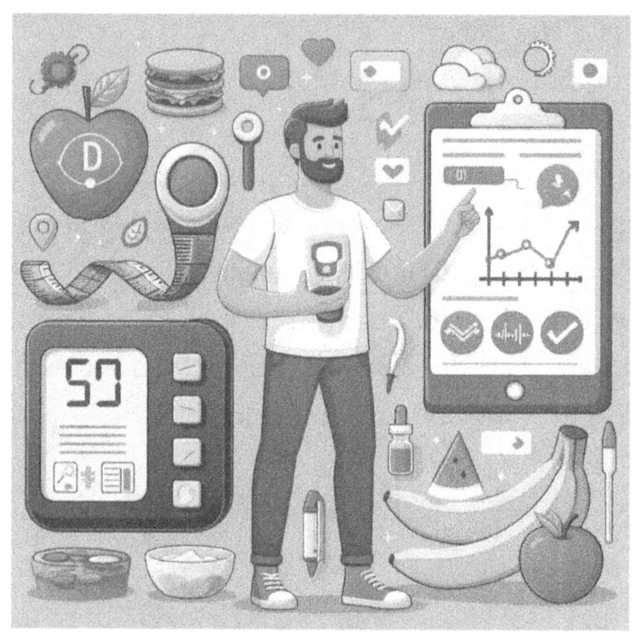

Monitoring and Adjusting Your Type 2 Diabetes Diet Plan

Chapter 10 : Monitoring and Adjusting Your Type 2 Diabetes Diet Plan

Monitoring and adjusting your type 2 diabetes diet plan is essential for achieving and maintaining optimal blood sugar control and overall health. This chapter explores the importance of regular monitoring, provides guidance on how to track dietary intake and blood sugar levels, and offers strategies for making adjustments to your diet plan as needed. By staying proactive and responsive to changes in your health and lifestyle, you can effectively manage your type 2 diabetes and minimize the risk of complications.

Importance of Monitoring:

- Regular monitoring of dietary intake and blood sugar levels is essential for understanding how different foods and lifestyle factors affect your diabetes management.
- Monitoring allows you to identify patterns, trends, and areas for improvement in your diet

and blood sugar control, empowering you to make informed decisions about your health.

- Monitoring provides valuable feedback that can help you assess the effectiveness of your current diet plan and make adjustments as needed to achieve your blood sugar goals.

Tracking Dietary Intake:

- Keep a food diary or use a mobile app to track your daily food intake, including portion sizes, carbohydrate content, and meal timing.
- Record not only what you eat but also how you feel before and after meals, as well as any symptoms or changes in blood sugar levels.
- Pay attention to patterns and trends in your eating habits, such as snacking behaviors, meal timing, and portion sizes, to identify areas for improvement.

Monitoring Blood Sugar Levels:

- Use a blood glucose meter to monitor your blood sugar levels regularly, as recommended by your healthcare provider.
- Keep a log of your blood sugar readings, including fasting levels, pre-meal levels,

post-meal levels, and bedtime levels, to track changes over time.

- Pay attention to factors that can affect blood sugar levels, such as exercise, medication, stress, illness, and changes in diet, and adjust your monitoring frequency accordingly.

Making Adjustments to Your Diet Plan:

- Use the information gathered from monitoring to identify patterns and trends in your blood sugar levels and dietary intake.
- Work with a registered dietitian or healthcare provider to make targeted adjustments to your diet plan, such as modifying portion sizes, carbohydrate content, meal timing, or food choices.
- Experiment with different meal plans, recipes, and eating patterns to find what works best for you and supports your blood sugar goals.
- Be patient and persistent in making changes to your diet plan, and monitor the effects on your blood sugar levels closely to assess their effectiveness.

Staying Flexible and Responsive:

- Diabetes management is not static, and your dietary needs may change over time due to factors such as age, weight, activity level, medication regimen, and overall health status.
- Stay flexible and open to making adjustments to your diet plan as needed to accommodate changes in your health, lifestyle, or preferences.
- Regularly revisit and review your diet plan with your healthcare team to ensure it remains aligned with your goals and supports your overall health and well-being.

By actively monitoring your dietary intake and blood sugar levels and making targeted adjustments to your diet plan as needed, you can effectively manage your type 2 diabetes and optimize your health outcomes. Remember to stay proactive, responsive, and engaged in your diabetes management to achieve long-term success.

Chapter 11: Overcoming Challenges and Staying Motivated

Successfully managing type 2 diabetes requires dedication, resilience, and ongoing motivation. This chapter addresses common challenges faced by individuals with type 2 diabetes and provides practical strategies for overcoming obstacles and staying motivated on the journey to better health. By recognizing and addressing challenges proactively and cultivating a positive mindset, individuals can overcome barriers to diabetes management and maintain long-term motivation for making healthy lifestyle choices.

Identifying Common Challenges:

- Lack of knowledge or understanding about diabetes management and healthy lifestyle practices.
- Difficulty adhering to dietary restrictions or making lasting changes to eating habits.

- Challenges with medication adherence, including remembering to take medications as prescribed and managing side effects.
- Emotional factors such as stress, depression, or anxiety, which can impact motivation and self-care behaviors.
- Social pressures or environmental factors that make it challenging to maintain healthy habits, such as social gatherings, holidays, or travel.

Strategies for Overcoming Challenges:

- Educate yourself about type 2 diabetes and healthy lifestyle practices through reliable sources of information, such as healthcare providers, diabetes educators, reputable websites, and support groups.
- Break down larger goals into smaller, achievable steps to make progress more manageable and sustainable.
- Seek support from healthcare professionals, family members, friends, or peer support groups who can provide encouragement, guidance, and accountability.

- Develop coping strategies for managing stress, such as mindfulness, relaxation techniques, exercise, or engaging in enjoyable activities.
- Plan ahead for challenging situations, such as social events or dining out, by making healthier food choices, bringing snacks or meals with you, or practicing portion control.
- Practice self-care and prioritize your physical, emotional, and mental well-being by engaging in activities that promote relaxation, stress relief, and positive self-talk.

Cultivating Motivation:

- Set specific, realistic goals for your diabetes management and overall health, and celebrate your progress along the way.
- Find your "why" – identify the reasons why managing your diabetes is important to you and use these motivations to fuel your commitment and perseverance.
- Focus on the benefits of healthy lifestyle choices, such as improved energy levels, better blood sugar control, reduced risk of complications, and enhanced overall quality of life.

- Surround yourself with positive influences and role models who inspire and support your health goals.
- Stay engaged and informed about new developments in diabetes management, treatment options, and research advances to maintain a sense of empowerment and hope for the future.

Embracing Resilience:

- Recognize that setbacks and challenges are a normal part of the diabetes journey and an opportunity for growth and learning.
- Practice resilience by bouncing back from setbacks, learning from mistakes, and adapting your approach as needed to overcome obstacles.
- Build resilience by developing coping skills, cultivating a positive outlook, and fostering a sense of self-efficacy and confidence in your ability to manage your diabetes effectively.

Celebrating Successes:

- Acknowledge and celebrate your achievements, no matter how small, as they represent progress toward your health goals.
- Keep a journal or log of your successes, milestones, and positive experiences to reflect on during challenging times and to remind yourself of how far you've come.
- Share your successes with others and use them as inspiration to motivate yourself and encourage others on their own diabetes journey.

By recognizing challenges, implementing effective strategies for overcoming obstacles, cultivating motivation, embracing resilience, and celebrating successes, individuals with type 2 diabetes can overcome barriers to diabetes management and stay motivated on their path to better health and well-being. Remember that managing diabetes is a journey, and every step forward is a victory worth celebrating

Thank you for choosing to purchase the "Dummies Type 2 Diabetes Diet Plan" book! Your decision to invest in your health and well-being is truly commendable. As an independent publisher, your support means the world to me, and I'm grateful for the opportunity to share valuable information that can positively impact your life.

Your feedback is incredibly valuable and helps me continue to improve the quality of my publications. If you found the "Dummies Type 2 Diabetes Diet Plan" book helpful, I would greatly appreciate it if you could take a moment to leave a review or share your thoughts. Your feedback not only assists me in refining future editions but also provides valuable insights for other individuals seeking reliable resources for managing type 2 diabetes.

Thank you once again for your support, and I hope the information provided in this book empowers you on your journey to better health and diabetes management.

Conclusion:

In the journey of managing type 2 diabetes, knowledge is power, and action is key. Throughout this book, we have explored various aspects of diabetes management, from understanding the different types of diabetes to implementing practical strategies for diet, exercise, and lifestyle changes. Here's a summary of the key takeaways:

Understanding Diabetes: We began by delving into the : Diet plays a crucial role in diabetes fundamentals of type 2 diabetes, including its definition, diagnosis criteria, risk factors, and prevalence. By understanding the nature of diabetes, individuals can make informed decisions about their health and take proactive steps to manage their condition effectively.

Dietary Management management, and we explored the importance of making healthy food choices, monitoring carbohydrate intake, and incorporating nutrient-dense foods into the diet. Emphasizing whole grains, lean proteins, fruits, vegetables, and healthy fats while limiting refined carbohydrates and added sugars can help stabilize blood sugar levels and promote overall health.

Exercise and Physical Activity: Regular exercise is essential for improving insulin sensitivity, lowering blood sugar levels, and reducing the risk of complications associated with type 2 diabetes. We discussed the benefits of aerobic exercise, strength training, flexibility, and balance exercises, as well as practical tips for incorporating physical activity into daily life.

Monitoring and Adjusting: Regular monitoring of blood sugar levels, dietary intake, and lifestyle factors is critical for assessing progress, identifying areas for improvement, and making necessary adjustments to the diabetes management plan. By staying proactive and responsive to changes in health and lifestyle, individuals can optimize their diabetes care and achieve better outcomes.

Overcoming Challenges and Staying Motivated: Managing type 2 diabetes can present various challenges, from dietary restrictions to emotional factors, but with resilience, support, and motivation, individuals can overcome obstacles and stay committed to their health goals. By cultivating a positive mindset, setting realistic goals, seeking support, and celebrating successes, individuals can navigate the ups and downs of diabetes management with confidence and determination.

In conclusion, managing type 2 diabetes is a multifaceted journey that requires knowledge, commitment, and perseverance. By taking proactive steps to understand the condition, make healthy lifestyle choices, and seek support when needed, individuals can empower themselves to live well with diabetes and enjoy a fulfilling life full of vitality and joy. Remember, you are not alone on this journey, and with the right tools and support, you can thrive with type 2 diabetes.

Thank you 💕